Against All Odds
Corall K. Holmes

Against All Odds

Against All Odds

Dedication

My grandmother "Queenie Turner" did so much for me during this whole process. She stayed with me during my hospital stay and was a lifesaver with my family. She bathed me, when I was too weak to bath myself. She had to help me to the bathroom and back. Many of the nights she was up with me, while I was sick, throwing up and in pain. She took on the mother role to my kids, because I was unable to be the mother I needed to be. She put everything, in her life, on hold just to take care of me.

My husband, Jimmy Holmes, had to go back to work at a grace period time and he travels out of town. He's such a great man and always has worked so hard to work to take care of all of us. Thank you for supporting me!

My kids Lee Trawick, Leonte Trawick, Madison London Holmes, Tyler Ashton Holmes, Jimmy Holmes, Ace Bryce Holmes and Jada Holmes.

Jada Holmes is my step daughter and she moved in with us 12/2013. She was a big help, as well, by her being a young lady. She was able to help my grandmother take care of me. She is very mature for her age and assisted me getting through the whole process.

Table of Contents

Chapter One

This Is Something Serious

I didn't realize what I was up against. I didn't know how to explain how I got here. I was living my life and moving right along and it seemed like I was hit out of nowhere. How could something so challenging come so unexpectedly and knock me off my feet? I was active, a go-getter, mom, wife, entrepreneur, student and minister. I had a lot going for me and bam, I was diagnosed with Sarcoidosis. What was this? I had never heard of such a disease. Something that I had never heard of came to visit me. When you are going through issues or suffering, they never announce themselves before striking. They just hit full force. They give you their best shot and now I was left to decipher the assault that had been launched against my body. I want to take you on a journey with me and let you hear how the power of God lifted me from a place of painful suffering to a place of experiencing life again, at its fullest potential.

Sarcoidosis is an inflammatory disease that affects multiple organs in the body, but mostly the lungs and lymph glands. In people with sarcoidosis, abnormal masses or nodules (called granulomas) consisting of inflamed tissues form in certain organs of the body. These granulomas may alter the normal structure and possibly the function of the affected organ(s).

The symptoms of sarcoidosis can vary greatly, depending on which organs are involved. Most patients initially complain of a persistent dry cough, fatigue, and shortness of breath. Other symptoms may include:

- Tender reddish bumps or patches on the skin.
- Red and teary eyes or blurred vision.
- Swollen and painful joints.
- Enlarged and tender lymph glands in the neck, armpits, and groin.
- Enlarged lymph glands in the chest and around the lungs.
- Hoarse voice.
- Pain in the hands, feet, or other bony areas due to the formation of cysts (an abnormal sac-like growth) in bones.
- Kidney stone formation.
- Enlarged liver.

- Development of abnormal or missed heart beats (arrhythmias), inflammation of the covering of the heart (pericarditis), or heart failure. Nervous system effects, including hearing loss, meningitis, seizures, or psychiatric disorders (for example, dementia, depression, psychosis).

In some people, symptoms may begin suddenly and/or severely and subside in a short period of time. Others may have no outward symptoms at all even though organs are affected. Still others may have symptoms that appear slowly and subtly, but which last or recur over a long time span. It normally occurs in people between the ages of 20 and 40 years of age. The disease is 10 to 17 times more common in African-Americans than in Caucasians. People of Scandinavian, German, Irish, or Puerto Rican origin are also more prone to the disease. It is estimated that up to four in 10,000 people in the U.S. have sarcoidosis. The exact cause of sarcoidosis is not known. It is a type of autoimmune disease associated with an abnormal immune response, but what triggers this response is uncertain. How sarcoidosis spreads from one part of the body to another is still being studied. Some of the diagnoses are not publicized, because there is not full knowledge about this disease. It is considered rare.

So, this is what hit me like a ton of bricks. I was about to travel down a road that I wasn't prepared for. I went from functioning at full capacity to feeling worthless, as a mother. I started to journal my days to remind me of my progress. I had to go through biopsies, MRI's, breathing treatments, x-ray's and on top of all of this experience pneumonia twice. I really felt like throwing in the towel. I had to remind myself who God was in my life. It would take me to:

Philippians 4:13

Philippians 4:13New King James Version (NKJV)

13 I can do all things through Christ[a] who strengthens me.

I had to learn to really hold onto God's unchanging hand and know that He is the same yesterday, today and forever. My mantra had officially become against all odds. This all started to happen around December 2013. I was in a very exciting time of life. I had just open my boutique and was hiring staff, stocking the store and preparing for business. I noticed that I was growing increasingly tired. By January 2014, I had developed a chronic cough. The cough dissipated, so I just assumed I had been hit with my yearly cold. It was cold and flu season.

But, by April, I started to begin coughing again. This time it was different. My chest was very tight. Nothing I took would cure it. By May, I had begun to vomit, every time I would eat. So, now my cough was elevating and I was just not feeling well. I felt very weak. This was about to give me a wakeup call. Even though I didn't understand, I had to hold on to this particular verse. This was about to reassure me of God's love and plans for me:

1 Corinthians 2:9New King James Version (NKJV)

⁹ But as it is written:

"Eye has not seen, nor ear heard,
Nor have entered into the heart of man
The things which God has prepared for those
who love Him."

Chapter Two

Dear Diary

In June 2014, I was closing the boutique, for the evening. My husband had come to visit and as we were walking to the car, I had shortness of breath, a cough and began to vomit blood. I immediately told him we needed to go to the emergency room. Something wasn't right! When I arrived, they did an x-ray. They had found spots on my lungs. Three doctors came in to talk to me. It was a frightening moment for me. They were making statements like they wanted to make sure this wasn't cancer and something very serious.

I was admitted that evening. I was sitting in my room crying and crying. It was so ironic, because when I got to my room there was a lady that was in the room with me. I couldn't see her, because the curtain was drawn, but I could hear her saying, "God has never failed me yet, so why would He start now?" This was all I needed to hear. I got out of bed, went in the restroom and wiped my tears away. Wow, God always speaks in our time of need. He is always there. Why was I afraid?

I had to remind myself that God is really for me.

Romans 8:28New King James Version (NKJV)

[28] And we know that all things work together for good to those who love God, to those who are the called according to *His* purpose.

This was where I had to abide, in Him. God was the only one who could stabilize my body and heal me. I had to put my full trust in Him and Him only. He has never let me down. There were times that I could not see my way out, but there was always a way prepared by Him.

I was prepped for a biopsy the next morning. They had to take tissue from my lungs. I was constantly on oxygen and I felt so weak. I was once again vomiting blood. 48 hours had gone by. The doctors had called a meeting, with me and my husband, to go over the results of testing. They informed me that this was not cancer, but I was diagnosed with Sarcoidosis. Because I was not familiar with this disease, I decided to journal what was happening in my life. I had to try to make sense of this. I had to start doing my own research, because the doctors were giving me vague answers.

I was told that the Sarcoidosis had rested in my lungs and bones. I had to have a cast on my left arms, due to the disease in my bones. I was hospitalized for three weeks. It was frustrating me, because I was so used to being on the go. Was I ever going to return to where I once was? I had to completely rely on God.

1 Peter 2:24New King James Version (NKJV)

24 who Himself bore our sins in His own body on the tree, that we, having died to sins, might live for righteousness—by whose stripes you were healed.

Healed, yes, I was going to decree, declare and prophesy over my life. I had to speak that I would live and live life more abundantly. I would not suffer isolation, rejection and relapse to a place that the enemy wanted me to visit. I had to dwell in the secret place of God, in order to remain focused on living.

Chapter Three

The Good, The Bad and The Ugly

I was placed on steroids. I was experiencing hot flashes, spasms, pains, insomnia and many other symptoms. Through all of this, my grandmother stayed and assisted. She was a life- saver. Between her and my husband, they were my life-lines to the outside world. I still had a business to run. I still had employees to pay. I couldn't let all of my hard work and dreams fall to the ground. I had to keep it afloat. My grandmother really took care of me. It was a great process. I had to deal with the hardships of financial strains and trying to meet all of the needs and demands that came with being a mom and business woman. When I came home from the hospital in July of 2014, I felt like I hit rock-bottom. I had feelings of depression and anxiety. What could be the good outcome of this? I was feeling afraid that I was going to die. I did not want to leave my beautiful children or beloved husband. We had overcome too much adversity together. I had to remain strong, just for them. I had to figure out my will. I just wanted everything to be in order, in my life. I know God does not give us the spirit of fear, but this was scary to me.

This would become my new theme verse, as many were sustaining me through the processing of the pain. But, I love this particular scripture, because it gives me such life.

Isaiah 41:10New King James Version (NKJV)

[10] Fear not, for I *am* with you;
Be not dismayed, for I *am* your God.
I will strengthen you,
Yes, I will help you,
I will uphold you with My righteous right hand.'

I had to face life head on and not waver, in the midst of adversity. In August of 2014, I was still battling depression and on top of this I was diagnosed with pneumonia again. I didn't think that I would be readmitted again. I thought I would've been cleared by now. June, July and August were my hardest months. I had to get out of this place. I started to lose my hair. I had long hair, before I was diagnosed and now I was bald. I had gain weight in excess of 60 pounds. I would look in the mirror and not recognize myself. Who was I turning into? I was so overwhelmed by this feeling. I would just sit and cry. It was so hard for me to deal with.

In September of 2014, I started having black-outs. I had to be referred to a heart specialist to ensure the Sarcoidosis never made it to my heart. I ended up in the hospital once again. I had to wear a heart monitor for a couples weeks and keep an eye on the movements, of my heart. I got to the point, where I said to myself, "I am going to take my life back." I began to decree and declare over my life that I would not remain here in the bad and ugly, but God wanted me to move into the good. I had to shift my mindset. Depression was not my destination. I had to get up and dust myself off, if I was going to see what God had planned for me.

Romans 12:2New King James Version (NKJV)

2 And do not be conformed to this world, but be transformed by the renewing of your mind, that you may prove what *is* that good and acceptable and perfect will of God.

I had to renew myself in God on a daily basis. This was the only way to make it. Outside noise will kill you. If you are ever going to make progress with God, you have to give Him access to your mind. I chose to live.

Chapter Four

Living At All Cost

You have to be willing to make necessary changes, if you are going to get your body in alignment and agreement with God's plan. In order for me to get better, I had to give it all to God. As soon as I did, I started to see the results. I had to be willing to change my diet and eat properly. I had to be willing to try to exercise. How many people may be in a better place physically, if they would just simply shift their habits with eating around. One or two small diet exchanges can begin to make a world of difference. For example, drinking water instead of soda will cause an almost immediate effect in your body. Discipline, will power, accountability, responsibility and the will to live are some phrases that come to mind, when wanting to be healthy and take care of your body. I didn't have a choice. I wanted to see the weight I had gained come off. I wanted to grow my hair back. I wanted my bone structure to be sound. I wanted my breathing regulated.

So, no more fast food. I was going to push myself to do I what I was able to do. I was not able to get on the tread mill, but I would force myself off of the couch. I started taking baby steps that would consistently begin to bring me back to health again. I knew God was faithful and He wanted me to live!

Psalm 46:10New King James Version (NKJV)

[10] Be still, and know that I *am* God;
I will be exalted among the nations,
I will be exalted in the earth.

I really believed this deep down in my heart and spirit. I was finally able to begin to see past the smoke-screen of depression and pain. I was officially going to make it. I was determined to outlive Sarcoidosis and win this battle. I had too much in me, going for me and promised to me to give up. I would hear, "You shall surely live and not die." Sometimes, it is not about dying in our physical body, but dying to the will of purpose. We get frustrated and don't understand set-backs, in our lives.

We can't comprehend the incapacitating things that come and knock us down and therefore, in trying to make sense of pain, we tend to prolong the process of God. He never intended for you to suffer forever. In 1 Peter 5:10, it says, "After you've suffered a little while." It doesn't say always suffering. We have to be able to flow in the timing of God. His thoughts towards us are great.

Jeremiah 29:11 New King James Version (NKJV)

11 For I know the thoughts that I think toward you, says the Lord, thoughts of peace and not of evil, to give you a future and a hope.

So, from this verse, I knew He expected me to reach my expected destination and that was not where I was, currently. He was going to fight my battle. I began to see a major turnaround in my life. I was able to come off of oxygen, my body levels began to balance and I was able to really start exercising. I found myself on the tread mill now, walking at a 3.8 fast speed. I was able to do that without taking a breathing treatment. I started to only need one treatment a week.

I am still taking medication for the disease, but my body have become regulated. I don't suffer from insomnia and body spasms. I am able to function very well. I was able to resume my business, being an incredible mom and loving wife. I didn't want to lose my family, while I felt like I was losing me. This was very important to me. I worked too hard to get to this place, for a disease called Sarcoidosis to take me out. The fighter that had been in me, since I was a little girl came alive and I decided to deliver a knockout punch to the enemy, once again. NO, you will not interrupt my ability to live in peace, joy and divine purpose. NO, you will not interrupt my rest. I will see the goodness of the Lord and walk in abundance and overflow.

I have to monitor my eating habits and they keep an eye on my heart. I had the will to fight this rare disease and lose the 50 pounds I had gained. I did it for me, my children and my husband. They needed me and I needed me. At the end of the day, God needed me to complete my earthly assignment.

I can stand flat-footed and surely say that I am an overcomer. You can overcome Sarcoidosis. You are not alone. You don't have to isolate yourself in this process. You are not rejected or abandoned. Get educated on the process. It may bring a drastic change, in your life, but you will make it through. We have to begin to educate people on the symptoms and difficulties of this disease.

The most amazing thing that happened through this whole process was that I got to see my father. I had not seen him in many, many years. I had been angry at him for so long, because he was absent in my life growing up. He had heard that I was sick, via Facebook. At my weakest point of life, my father showed up. He sat in the hospital room for an entire day. God was beginning to repair the breach and brokenness that had been in place for so many years. We often don't understand why. But, God has everything under control. He orchestrates things so perfectly, in our lives that we can't help but to give Him the glory. He is an amazing God. I had to let my past pain and anger go. I had to forgive and this helped in my process of healing.

I have been very healthy for the last five months. I have gotten back on my feet completely. I am determined to educate others concerning what I went through. I want the Sarcoidosis community and sufferers to know that it is not the end of life, as they know it. You can take your right to live back. Stand for you, your family and your purpose. I stand with my boxing gloves on and say proudly, "Against all odds, I have made it!"

Contact Information

To book Corall K. Holmes to speak at your upcoming event, you may go to:

www.corallkholmes.com

www.gachristianboutique.com

or email:

gachristianboutique@gmail.com